NUTRITION FOR LIFE

A COMPREHENSIVE GUIDE TO NOURISHING

YOUR BODY AND MIND

AHMED .R

Contents

CHAPTER ONE

INTRODUCTION

In today's hectic world, when time is scarce and convenience frequently takes precedence over health, keeping a nutritious and well-balanced diet can seem like an overwhelming task. Nonetheless, the value of a healthy diet cannot be emphasized in the midst of the confusion of modern life. It is the foundation that supports both our mental and physical health.

Welcome to "Nutrition for Life: A Comprehensive Guide to Nourishing Your Body and Mind." We will be exploring the significant effects that nutrition has on all facets of our life as we work through the intricacies of nutrition. Our diet has a significant impact on our health, energy levels, cognitive function, and even emotional state, influencing everything from our daily interactions to the molecular level.

This book is not your typical diet guide or compilation of dos and don'ts. Rather, it is a comprehensive investigation of nutrition as a way of life—a quest for knowledge, self-awareness, and empowerment. This guide includes helpful insights, doable tactics, and evidence-based knowledge to help you make informed decisions and develop a long-lasting relationship with food, regardless of your level of experience with nutrition.

We'll dispel myths, examine new developments, and sort through a deluge of nutritional data to extract the key ideas that support a nutritious diet in these pages. Every chapter is designed to give you the information and resources you need to confidently navigate the complexity of nutrition, from the advantages of whole foods to the function of micronutrients and the influence of dietary patterns on the prevention of chronic diseases.

Still, this book offers much more than a guide to physical well-being. We'll also examine the complex relationships that exist between mental health and nutrition, including how our diet affects our mood, mental clarity, and general resilience. We may use food to create a healthy and vibrant existence by realizing the close connection between mental health and nutrition.

"Nutrition for Life" is fundamentally a celebration of the amazing potential for health transformation that everyone of us possesses.

The Significance of Diet in Overall Health and Well-Being

In order to promote general health and wellness at every stage of life, nutrition is essential. It includes eating a diet that is well-balanced and rich in the vitamins, minerals, and other bioactive substances that are vital for the body to function at its best. The following main ideas emphasize how crucial diet is to overall health and wellbeing:

Promotes Growth and Development: As it offers the nutrients required for growth, development, and cognitive function, a healthy diet is important for kids and teenagers. During these phases, a healthy diet rich in protein, vitamins, and minerals promotes both mental and physical development.

Maintains Healthy Body Weight: By giving the proper quantity of calories and nutrients without going overboard, a balanced diet aids in keeping a healthy body weight. Eating foods high in nutrients, like fruits, vegetables, whole grains, and lean meats, can help avoid obesity and its associated chronic illnesses.

Prevents Chronic Diseases: Heart disease, diabetes, and some forms of cancer are among the chronic diseases that nutrition is known to help avoid. Inflammation, oxidative stress, and maintaining ideal blood pressure and cholesterol levels can all be decreased by eating a diet high in fruits, vegetables, whole grains, and healthy fats.

Supports Immune Function: A robust immune system depends on appropriate diet. Vitamins A, C, D, E, zinc, and selenium are among the nutrients that are essential for boosting immune system performance and lowering infection risk. Eating a range of foods high in nutrients fortifies the body's defenses against disease and speeds up healing after illness.

Enhances Mental Health: An increasing amount of research is showing a connection between mental health and diet. Eating a diet high in fruits, vegetables, whole grains, and omega-3 fatty acids may enhance mood and cognitive performance while reducing the risk of anxiety and depression.

Boosts Athletic Performance: In order to feed their bodies and maximize performance, athletes need to eat a healthy diet. Before, during, and after exercise, consuming enough carbs, proteins, and water supports muscle repair and recovery, boosts energy levels, and increases strength and endurance.

Enhances Lifespan and Well-Being: Maintaining a nutritious diet and way of living can have a big impact on lifespan and well-being. People can live longer, healthier lives when they follow a balanced diet, which lowers their risk of chronic diseases and improves their general well-being when combined with regular exercise, enough sleep, and stress management.

diet plays a critical role in both obtaining and preserving good health and wellness. People may nourish their bodies, avoid disease, and live better overall by choosing foods wisely and developing good eating habits.

The Basics of Nutrition

It is crucial to comprehend the principles of nutrition in order to make well-informed food decisions and preserve general health and wellbeing. The following are the main elements of nutrition:

The macronutrients

Carbs: The body uses carbohydrates as its main energy source. They are present in foods including grains, fruits, vegetables, and legumes and consist of sugars, starches, and fiber.

Proteins: Building and mending tissues as well as performing a number of other biological tasks depend on proteins. Meat, poultry, fish, dairy products, eggs, legumes, nuts, and seeds are all excellent sources of protein.

Fats: Fats aid in the body's absorption of specific vitamins, support cell growth, and supply energy. Avocados, almonds, seeds, olive oil, fatty fish, and plant-based oils are examples of healthy fat sources.

Small-scale nutrients:

Vitamins: Vitamins are necessary micronutrients with specialized roles in immune system function, metabolism, and bone health, among other body processes. They can be found in many different foods, such as dairy products, fruits, vegetables, and foods that have been fortified.

Minerals: Minerals are essential for a number of physiological functions, such as neuron function, fluid balance, and bone health. Minerals include calcium, magnesium, iron, potassium, and zinc.

Whole grains, dairy products, nuts, seeds, and leafy greens are good sources of these nutrients.

Aqua:

Water is essential for carrying nutrients, removing waste, controlling body temperature, and staying hydrated. It is advised to drink enough water each day, which can be obtained from beverages and foods high in water content, such as fruits and vegetables.

Nutritional Guidelines:

Dietary guidelines offer suggestions for wholesome eating habits that are supported by scientific data. Generally speaking, these recommendations place an emphasis on eating a range of foods high in nutrients, avoiding added sweets, saturated fats, and sodium, and regulating calorie consumption in relation to physical activity.

Density of nutrients:

The quantity of nutrients (such as vitamins, minerals, and fiber) in relation to the number of calories in a food is referred to as its nutritional density. Selecting foods high in nutrients, such as whole grains, fruits, vegetables, lean meats, and healthy fats, will help you make the most of every calorie you eat.

A well-rounded diet

In order to meet nutritional needs, a balanced diet consists of a range of foods from all food categories in the right amounts. This lowers the risk of vitamin shortages and chronic diseases while promoting general health.

Personal Requirements:

A number of variables, including age, gender, body size, degree of exercise, health, and metabolic rate, affect nutritional needs. Dietary decisions must be customized to each person's requirements and tastes.

People can optimize their nutrient intake, make educated dietary decisions, and promote their general health and well-being by knowing these basic principles of nutrition.

Comprehending Dietary Guidelines

It is essential to comprehend dietary recommendations in order to encourage wholesome eating practices and general wellbeing. Here's a summary of the main points:

A. International and National Dietary Guidelines:

both domestic and global health institutions, including the U.S. Dietary guidelines are based on scientific research and are released by the Department of Agriculture (USDA), the World Health Organization (WHO), and the European Food Safety Authority (EFSA).

Usually, these suggestions include instructions for eating a balanced diet that minimizes the risk of chronic diseases and offers necessary nutrients.

They frequently include suggested intake ranges for micronutrients (vitamins, minerals) and macronutrients (carbs, proteins, and fats) depending on factors including age, gender, and degree of exercise.

B. Models of the Food Pyramid and Plate: Recommendations for a Balanced Diet

Food pyramids and plate models give advice on portion sizes and food selections for a balanced diet by visually representing dietary requirements.

The conventional food pyramid divides food groups into sections and suggests how much of each group should be consumed.

In order to depict a balanced meal composition, the more recent food plate model separates a plate into parts that correspond to several food groups, such as fruits, vegetables, grains, and proteins.

These models stress the significance of eating a range of foods high in nutrients and minimizing the consumption of harmful options such as processed foods and sugary snacks.

C. Useful Hints for Applying Dietary Guidelines in Everyday Situations:

Make a weekly meal plan that consists of a range of nutrient-dense foods from all the food groups.

Read labels: Take note of the nutritional information on product labels to help you make wise decisions regarding the ingredients in packaged goods.

Use smaller bowls and plates to regulate portion sizes and prevent overindulging.

Cook at home: To have more control over the ingredients and cooking techniques, prepare meals at home with whole, fresh ingredients.

Incorporate fruits and veggies: To enhance consumption of important vitamins, minerals, and fiber, try to fill half of your plate with fruits and vegetables at each meal.

Reduce the amount of processed foods you eat. Processed foods are high in sodium, bad fats, and added sugars.

Remain hydrated by limiting your intake of sugar-filled beverages and drinking lots of water throughout the day.

Be aware of your eating habits: To prevent emotional or distracted eating, be aware of your hunger and fullness cues and engage in mindful eating.

Through comprehension and application of dietary recommendations in everyday life, people can enhance their nutritional intake, choose better foods, and lower their chance of developing chronic diseases linked to diet.

The Relationship Between Health and Nutrition

There is a complex relationship between diet and health that affects both mental and physical well-being in different ways. Here is a look at some important links:

A. Avoiding Chronic Illnesses with a Nutritious Diet:

In order to prevent chronic conditions including heart disease, diabetes, obesity, and some types of cancer, nutrition is essential.

Eating a well-balanced diet full of whole grains, fruits, vegetables, lean meats, and healthy fats supplies antioxidants and other vital nutrients that help lower oxidative stress, inflammation, and other risk factors linked to chronic illnesses.

Diets rich in fruits and vegetables, for instance, have been associated with a lower risk of stroke and heart disease, while meals high in fiber can help control blood sugar levels and lessen the risk of type 2 diabetes.

B. Increasing Immune Response and Promoting General Well-Being:

CHAPTER TWO

A strong immune system, which protects the body from diseases and infections, depends on proper nutrition.

The immune system depends on several nutrients, which can be found in a range of foods such as fruits, vegetables, dairy products, lean meats, and vitamins A, C, D, E, zinc, and selenium.

Eating a well-balanced diet full of nutrients that enhance the immune system can help the body fight off infections and lower the risk of getting sick with the flu and colds.

C. Enhancing Mental Well-Being and Cognitive Ability with Appropriate Diet:

Cognitive function and mental health are also greatly impacted by nutrition.

An increased risk of depression, anxiety, and cognitive decline has been linked to diets heavy in processed foods, refined sugars, and unhealthy fats.

In contrast, studies have shown that eating a diet high in fruits, vegetables, whole grains, and omega-3 fatty acids improves mental health, elevates mood, and lowers the risk of cognitive decline.

Certain nutrients are especially crucial for brain health and cognitive function, such as the omega-3 fatty acids found in fatty fish and the B vitamins found in leafy greens and whole grains.

In conclusion, the relationship between diet and health is clear given its ability to prevent chronic illnesses, strengthen the immune system, promote general wellness, and enhance mental and cognitive performance. A balanced diet that emphasizes foods high in nutrients can help people improve their health and well-being in many areas of their lives.

Putting Together a Healthful Plate

Choosing a range of nutrient-rich foods in the right amounts to make balanced meals is the foundation of creating a healthy plate. The following methods will help you construct a plate that is healthful:

Arrange Fruits and Vegetables on Half of Your Plate:

Try to fill half of your plate with vegetables and fruits. To make sure you get a diverse spectrum of vitamins, minerals, and antioxidants, choose a variety of colors and varieties.

To optimize nutrient intake, include fresh fruits and berries along with cooked and raw veggies.

Incorporate Lean Proteins:

On your plate, place a lean protein source such as fish, chicken, tofu, beans, lentils, or lean meat portions.

To cut back on extra fats and calories, choose protein sources that are baked, roasted, or grilled rather than fried or highly processed.

Add Whole Grains:

To get fiber, vitamins, and minerals, choose whole grains like brown rice, quinoa, barley, whole wheat pasta, or whole grain bread.

Steer clear of refined grains, which have had their nutrients removed through processing, such as white bread and rice.

Add Good Fats:

Include foods like nuts, seeds, avocados, olive oil, and fatty fish like trout or salmon in your diet as sources of healthful fats.

Reduce your intake of processed meals, fried foods, and high-fat meats since they include saturated and trans fats, which raise your risk of heart disease.

Monitor Portion Measurements:

Pay attention to portion proportions to prevent overindulging. To help you manage portion sizes, use smaller bowls and plates and pay attention to your body's signals of hunger and fullness.

To guarantee a balanced diet free of excess calories, pay attention to the portion sizes that are suggested for the various food categories.

Limit Sodium and Added Sugars:

Reduce your intake of foods and drinks with a lot of added sugar, such as processed snacks, sweetened drinks, and desserts.

Limit your consumption of sodium by selecting low- or no-sodium foods and enhancing food flavor with citrus, herbs, and spices rather than salt.

Maintain Hydration:

In order to maintain proper biological functioning and stay hydrated, don't forget to drink lots of water throughout the day.

Alcohol and sugar-filled drinks should be avoided as they might cause dehydration and empty calorie intake.

By adhering to these recommendations and assembling a nutritious plate comprising an assortment of nutrient-dense foods, you can bolster general health and wellness while relishing delectable and fulfilling meals.

The Value of Well-Composed Meals and Snacks

Maintaining energy levels, promoting general health, and avoiding overeating all depend on eating balanced meals and snacks. This is the reason they matter:

Sustained Energy Levels: The body requires a combination of macronutrients (proteins, fats, and carbohydrates) and micronutrients (vitamins and minerals) for balanced meals and snacks in order to perform at its best. Different rates of nutrient absorption and breakdown enable these nutrients to support sustained energy levels throughout the day.

Control of Blood Sugar: Consuming well-balanced meals and snacks helps control blood sugar levels, avoiding the spikes and crashes that can cause exhaustion, mood changes, and cravings. Stable blood sugar levels are promoted by consuming meals and snacks that include lean proteins, healthy fats, and fiber-rich carbohydrates. This slows down the absorption of sugar into the bloodstream.

Supports Weight Management: By offering a variety of nutrients that encourage fullness, balanced meals and snacks can help control hunger and stop overeating. Particularly fiber and protein are well known for their capacity to keep you feeling full and content in between meals, which lowers the chance of consuming too many calories.

Nutrient Absorption: You may make sure your body gets the vital vitamins, minerals, and other components it needs for optimum health by eating a range of nutrient-rich foods in balanced meals and snacks. Nutrient utilization and absorption are maximized by a balanced diet, as different nutrients complement one another.

Promotes General Health: By offering the nutrients required for healthy bodily processes, such as immune response, digestion, metabolism, and tissue repair, balanced meals and snacks promote general health and wellbeing. A diet high in a variety of nutrients derived from whole foods can promote longevity and lower the risk of chronic illnesses.

Improves Mental Performance: Clear thinking and proper nourishment are necessary for cognitive performance. Focus, concentration, and mood can all be enhanced by eating balanced meals and snacks that include nutrients that support the brain, such as antioxidants, omega-3 fatty acids, and B vitamins.

Encourages Mindful Eating: Including balanced meals and snacks in your daily routine helps you avoid becoming overly dependent on processed foods or eating a lot of empty-calorie snacks. It also encourages mindful eating. Making better dietary choices can also involve prepping and planning balanced meals and snacks.

healthy eating habits, blood sugar regulation, weight control, general health promotion, improved mental function, and energy maintenance are all facilitated by eating balanced meals and snacks. Nutrient-rich foods are important, and you may maximize your health and well-being by making them a regular part of your diet.

Including Color and Variety in Your Diet

In addition to being aesthetically pleasing, adding diversity and color to your diet is key to guaranteeing that you get a wide range of nutrients that are necessary for optimum health. The following explains the significance of variety and color as well as how to include them in your meals:

Nutrient Diversity: Unique combinations of vitamins, minerals, antioxidants, and phytochemicals can be found in a variety of fruits, vegetables, grains, proteins, and fats. You can guarantee that you get a broad spectrum of nutrients required for different body functions by eating a variety of foods.

Health Benefits: The many colors seen in fruits and vegetables correspond to distinct phytochemicals, each of which has unique health advantages. Lycopene, for instance, is found in red fruits and vegetables like tomatoes and red bell peppers and may help lower the risk of heart disease and some types of cancer.

Antioxidant Protection: Rich in antioxidants, fruits and vegetables with vibrant colors help lower inflammation and fight oxidative stress in the body. Consuming a wide range of vibrant produce can boost your immunity and reduce your chance of developing long-term health issues.

Eating a vibrant and aesthetically pleasing meal can increase hunger stimulation and make eating more pleasurable. In addition to keeping meals interesting, variety in hues and textures might motivate you to try new foods.

Disease Prevention: Studies have shown a decreased risk of chronic illnesses like heart disease, diabetes, obesity, and some types of cancer in those who eat a diet high in whole grains, lean meats, and colorful fruits and vegetables. Including a range of colors in your diet contributes to your general health and wellbeing.

The following advice can help you add diversity and color to your diet:

Eat the Rainbow: Make an effort to incorporate a variety of colored fruits and vegetables into your meals and snacks. Pick purple eggplant, blueberries, green spinach, orange carrots, yellow bell peppers, and red tomatoes, for instance.

Try New Foods: To add diversity to your diet, try a range of fruits, vegetables, grains, legumes, and proteins. To find novel and unusual ingredients, visit ethnic grocery stores or farmers' markets.

Vary Your Cooking Techniques: To bring out the flavors and textures of fruits and vegetables, try preparing them in a variety of ways, including raw, steamed, roasted, grilled, or sautéed. Foods with varying hues and nutritional values can also be enhanced by different cooking techniques.

Legumes and Whole Grains: To vary your sources of carbohydrates and proteins, include legumes like beans, lentils, and chickpeas as well as whole grains like brown rice, quinoa, barley, and whole wheat pasta.

Add Herbs and Spices: You may flavor and color your food without adding extra sodium or calories by using herbs, spices, and condiments. Try experimenting with spices like paprika, cinnamon, and turmeric, and fresh herbs like parsley, cilantro, and basil.

You can enjoy a wide range of nutrients, flavors, and health benefits while increasing general well-being and meal pleasure by making variety and color a priority in your diet.

Portion control and Conscious Consumption

A healthy relationship with food requires portion control and mindful eating techniques, which also help to prevent overeating by raising awareness of hunger and fullness cues. Here's how to make mindful eating and portion control a part of your everyday routine:

Consider Portion Sizes:

To estimate portion sizes, look for visual cues. One portion of protein, for instance, should be roughly the size of your palm; one serving of carbohydrates, approximately the size of your fist; and one serving of fats, approximately the size of your thumb.

By reading nutrition labels and, where necessary, using measuring cups, spoons, or a kitchen scale, you can become familiar with typical portion proportions.

Eating straight out of big packages or containers should be avoided since this could result in thoughtless overindulgence. Rather, before eating, divide portions into a plate or dish.

Eat Often and Consciously:

Set aside regular times for meals, and make an effort to avoid distractions like TV watching or phone browsing. Pay attention to all of your senses while you eat, including the flavor, texture, and aroma of your food.

Chew your food slowly and deeply, enjoying every bite. You can identify feelings of fullness and avoid overeating by eating slowly.

Observe the signals your body sends when it is hungry or full. Eat only until you are full, even if there is food left on your plate. Eat when you are hungry.

Use portion control strategies:

Reduce the size of your dishes, plates, and utensils to help you eat less and avoid overindulging. Smaller dishware tends to make individuals eat less, according to research.

Place non-starchy veggies on half of your plate, lean protein on one quarter, and whole grains or starchy vegetables on the other quarter. By using a balanced approach, you can be confident that you are getting plenty of different nutrients without going overboard with any one food group.

Take note of the liquid calories found in liquids such as juice, soda, and alcoholic beverages. Choose low-calorie liquids like water or herbal tea, and avoid high-calorie drinks that may lead to overindulgence in calories.

Pay Attention to Your Body:

Prior to, during, and after eating, pay attention to your body's indications of hunger and fullness. Eat when your body tells you to and stop eating when you're full, even if there's food left over.

Be mindful of the emotional and environmental cues such as stress, boredom, or the appearance of appetizing foods that can lead to overeating. Seek out other coping mechanisms or divert your attention from eating desires.

Exercise appreciation and gratitude:

Practice being thankful for the food you eat and the health benefits it offers your body. Give thanks for the work that went into making your meals by taking a moment to enjoy their tastes, textures, and colors.

You may prevent overeating, foster general wellbeing, and create a healthier connection with food by adopting mindful eating habits and portion control into your daily routine. Additionally, by following these guidelines, you'll be able to enjoy your meals more and feel content with smaller servings.

Consumption of Food Throughout Life

Due to several factors like growth, development, metabolism, and lifestyle changes, there are differences in nutrition needs during the lifespan. An outline of dietary needs and factors to take into account at various life phases is provided below:

Early life (0–12 months):

For the first six months of life, an infant can get all the nutrients they need from breast milk or formula, with breast milk being the best option when it is available.

Around six months of age, supplementary foods are usually introduced. Pureed fruits, vegetables, meats, and grains are progressively added, with iron-fortified cereals serving as the foundation.

It is recommended to breastfeed during the first year of life, and even longer if the mother and child so want.

Early Life (ages 1 to 5):

Preschoolers and toddlers require more energy and nutrients to sustain their continued growth and development.

The provision of a range of nutrient-dense foods, including as fruits, vegetables, whole grains, lean proteins, and dairy products, should be prioritized.

To suit their tiny stomachs and erratic appetites, serve them modest, frequent meals and snacks.

To promote healthy eating habits, encourage self-feeding and experimentation with various textures and flavors.

Children in school (6–12 years old):

Balanced meals and snacks are necessary for school-age children to promote growth, physical exercise, and cognitive function.

CHAPTER THREE

Promote a varied diet that is high in whole grains, fruits, vegetables, lean meats, low-fat dairy products, and other nutrients.

Children should be taught the value of balanced meals, portion sizes, and the role that nutrients play in fostering health and wellbeing.

Involve kids in meal planning, grocery shopping, and food preparation to encourage good eating habits.

Teenage years (13–18):

Teenagers grow and develop quickly, so they need to consume more iron, calcium, protein, and energy.

Promote the eating of meals high in nutrients to help you fulfill your increased energy needs and maintain a healthy weight.

Stress the value of eating well-balanced meals, getting regular exercise, and drinking enough water.

Teach teenagers about the possible effects of food on long-term health outcomes, bone health, and hormonal changes.

Adulthood (ages 19–64):

The goal of maintaining a balanced diet that supports general health and well-being and satisfies nutrient needs is to concentrate on this during adulthood.

Place a strong emphasis on eating a variety of whole foods, such as fruits, vegetables, whole grains, lean meats, and healthy fats.

Keep an eye on portion sizes, cut back on processed foods and added sugars, and make regular exercise a part of your everyday routine.

Take care of your body's unique dietary requirements depending on your lifestyle, chronic illnesses, pregnancy, and lactation.

Senior Citizens (65 and older):

Due to variables like diminished metabolism, decreased appetite, altered digestion, and long-term medical issues, older persons may have shifting dietary demands.

To guarantee sufficient consumption of vital nutrients while controlling calorie intake, concentrate on nutrient-dense foods.

Because older persons may be more susceptible to dehydration, pay attention to their hydration levels.

Think about the significance of protein for maintaining and repairing muscles, fiber for digestive health, and calcium and vitamin D for bone health.

Promote social interaction and regular exercise to enhance general health and wellbeing in older adults.

All things considered, diet is extremely important for maintaining health and wellbeing throughout life. People can maximize their health and quality of life by attending to unique nutritional demands and encouraging good eating habits at every stage of life.

Dietary Guidelines for Particular Populations

Addressing the particular nutritional requirements and considerations of particular groups based on variables including age, health conditions, cultural origins, and lifestyle choices is known as nutrition for special populations. An outline of nutrition-related concerns for several special populations is provided below:

Women who are expecting or nursing:

Women who are pregnant or nursing require more nutrients to support both the growth and development of the fetus and the production of milk.

Enough consumption of protein, calcium, iron, omega-3 fatty acids, folate, and other vital nutrients should be stressed.

Promote the eating of a range of nutrient-dense foods, such as whole grains, dairy products, fruits, vegetables, and lean meats.

Inform pregnant women about foods to stay away from, like raw seafood, unpasteurized dairy products, and some mercury-high fish varieties.

Young Children and Infants:

For the purpose of promoting growth, development, and immune system function, infants and early children have specific nutritional demands.

For the first year of life, breast milk or formula offers the best nourishment; starting at the age of six months, complementary foods are gradually introduced.

To encourage good eating habits from an early age, encourage the introduction of a range of foods, textures, and flavors that are high in nutrients.

When introducing new foods, keep an eye out for any indications of food allergies or intolerances and seek medical advice if you have any concerns.

Youngsters and Teenagers:

The nutritional requirements of children and adolescents are higher in order to support growth, physical activity, and cognitive development.

Stress the value of eating a range of fruits, vegetables, whole grains, lean meats, and dairy products in your meals and snacks.

Teach kids and teenagers the value of sensible eating practices, portion management, and the part that nutrients play in fostering health and wellbeing.

In a helpful and nonjudgmental approach, address nutrition-related difficulties such as finicky eating, disordered eating patterns, and body image issues.

Senior Citizens:

Older persons may have different nutritional demands because of things like slower metabolism, less hunger, altered digestion, and long-term medical issues.

To guarantee sufficient intake of vital nutrients while controlling calorie intake, promote the consumption of foods high in nutrients.

Address certain dietary issues that older persons often face, such as malnutrition, dehydration, and nutrient shortages.

Think about the significance of protein for maintaining and repairing muscles in older adulthood, fiber for digestive health, and calcium and vitamin D for bone health.

Active People and Athletes:

The energy and nutritional requirements of athletes and active people are higher in order to support physical activity, training, and recuperation.

Stress the importance of consuming protein for muscle growth and repair, carbs for energy, and water for hydration.

Promote a diet that is well-balanced and rich in a range of nutrients, such as fruits, vegetables, whole grains, lean meats, and healthy fats.

For the best results and recuperation, take into account particular nutrition factors including hydration tactics, timing of nutrients, and nutrition before and after exercise.

There may be particular dietary guidelines or advice for those with long-term illnesses or ailments depending on their circumstances.

Create a customized nutrition plan in collaboration with a medical professional or registered dietitian that takes into account each person's dietary preferences, lifestyle choices, and health requirements.

Stress the significance of controlling blood pressure, cholesterol, blood sugar, and other health indicators with food, exercise, and medication.

Inform them about the importance of diet in controlling their illness and lowering the chance of complications.

Minorities in culture and ethnicity:

Minority cultures and ethnic groups may follow different eating customs, traditions, and dietary preferences, which can affect how much nutrients they consume.

Incorporate traditional meals and recipes into nutrition teaching and counseling programs while honoring ethnic uniqueness.

Think about how social, religious, and cultural norms may influence dietary preferences, access to wholesome foods, and behaviors linked to nutrition.

Work together with local resources, cultural organizations, and leaders in the community to offer nutrition instruction and support that is appropriate for the local culture.

In general, nutrition for special populations entails modifying dietary guidelines and interventions to take into account the unique requirements, inclinations, and difficulties of various groups. Healthcare practitioners and nutrition specialists can advance health equity, increase the well-being of specific groups, and improve health outcomes by adopting a tailored approach to nutrition treatment.

Comprehending Nutrition Labels and Making Well-Informed Decisions

Comprehending food labels is essential to make knowledgeable decisions about the meals we eat. Here is an explanation of the main elements on food labels and how to utilize them to help you choose healthier options:

Serving Size: All additional nutritional information is dependent on the serving size specified on the label, so pay close attention to it. To be sure you're getting enough nutrients, check the serving size against how much you usually consume.

Calories: The quantity of energy that a food item has is indicated by the number of calories per serving. Pay attention to your overall caloric intake and portion sizes, particularly if you're attempting to control your weight.

Nutrient Content: The amounts of different macronutrients (such fat, carbs, and protein) and micronutrients (like vitamins and minerals) in each serving are usually listed on food labels. Choose foods high in nutrients and low in salt, saturated fats, and added sugars.

% Daily Value (%DV): Based on a diet of 2,000 calories, the %DV shows how much a serving of an item contributes to your daily recommended intake of each nutrient. To assess the nutritional content of various foods and make well-informed decisions about their nutritional worth, use the %DV.

Ingredients List: The ingredients list, which is arranged in decreasing weight order, contains details about each food product's constituent parts. Start your search for products with identifiable ingredients and whole foods at the top of the list. Stay away from anything that include preservatives, artificial additives, or added sugars.

Health Claims: Food labels may contain symbols or health claims that highlight a product's high fiber content, low fat content, or suitability as a source of specific vitamins or minerals. Always study the entire nutrition label to determine the food's overall nutritional quality and be wary of marketing claims.

Allergen Information: To assist those with food allergies or sensitivities in avoiding possible triggers, food labels are required to disclose common allergens, including milk, eggs, wheat, soy, peanuts, tree nuts, fish, and shellfish.

Expiration Date or Best Before Date: Verify the food product's freshness and safety by paying attention to its expiration or best before date. Foods should be consumed before they expire to ensure maximum quality and safety.

Focus on choosing complete, minimally processed foods that are high in nutrients and low in added sugars, harmful fats, and sodium when using food labels to make educated decisions. To promote general health and wellbeing, include a range of fruits, vegetables, whole grains, lean meats, and healthy fats in your diet.

Finding Sugars, Fats, and Additives That Are Hidden

It might be difficult to recognize hidden sugars, fats, and additives in food items, but doing so is crucial if you want to make healthy eating decisions. The following advice will help you recognize and consume fewer of these hidden ingredients:

Examine ingredient lists: Since ingredients are listed by weight in descending order, the product's bulk is comprised of the first few ingredients. If you're looking for hidden sugars in an ingredient list, look for terms like "sugar," "high-fructose corn syrup," "corn syrup," "honey," "molasses," "agave nectar," "sucrose," and other sweeteners.

Watch Out for Other Names: Sugar can be found under a variety of names, such as fructose, glucose, cane sugar, beet sugar, fruit juice concentrate, maltose, lactose, and many more. Whenever you read ingredient lists, keep these alternate names in mind.

Examine Nutrition Labels: Take note of the total sugar amount specified on the label. Remember that natural and added sugars are not distinguished by the % Daily Value (%DV), so it is important to check the ingredient list for clarification.

Be Wary of Low-Fat or Fat-Free goods: To improve flavor and texture, some low-fat or fat-free goods may include additional sugars or other additives. To evaluate the overall nutritional quality of these goods, review the nutrition label and ingredient list.

Look for Hidden Fats: Under many other names, including trans fats, partially hydrogenated oils, hydrogenated oils, palm oil, coconut oil, and various emulsifiers and stabilizers, fats can also be found in processed foods. Products with these substances should be avoided since they may increase consumption of harmful fats.

Preservatives (such BHA and BHT) and artificial colors, tastes, sweeteners (including aspartame, saccharin, and sucralose), and other chemical additives should all be avoided. These components are frequently found in processed and packaged meals, and they may pose health hazards.

CHAPTER FOUR

Select Whole Foods: Since they are less likely to include unrecognized added sugars, fats, or chemicals, choose whole, minimally processed foods wherever available. Nutritious foods include fruits, vegetables, whole grains, lean meats, nuts, seeds, and legumes. They also don't contain added sweets or bad fats.

Cook Meals at Home: Making meals at home gives you complete control over the products you use and lowers your exposure to additives, hidden sugars, and fats that are frequently found in processed foods and meals from restaurants.

You may enhance the quality of your diet overall and promote better health outcomes by raising your awareness of the hidden sugars, fats, and additives in food products and making deliberate decisions to limit your intake of these elements.

Advice for Efficient Meal Planning and Grocery Purchasing

Meal planning and grocery shopping are crucial for preserving a balanced diet, cutting down on food waste, and saving time. The following advice may help you make better meal plans and purchase more wisely:

Enumerate the groceries:

Make a list of the things you'll need based on your weekly meal plans before you go shopping.

To make your trip through the shop more effective, arrange your list according to food groups (such as produce, dairy, grains, and proteins).

Arrange Your Meals in Advance:

Spend some time organizing your weekly menu, covering breakfast, lunch, dinner, and snacks.

When organizing meals, take into account your nutritional objectives, dietary preferences, and schedule.

For a balanced diet, try to eat a range of foods from various dietary categories.

Examine the sales flyers and inventory:

Make a list of everything you currently own so you don't buy duplicates.

Examine discounts and sales fliers to find affordable options for basic goods and foods.

Choose Foods High in Nutrients:

Give nutrient-dense foods like fruits, vegetables, whole grains, lean meats, and healthy fats priority in your diet.

Whenever possible, choose whole, fresh foods over packaged and processed ones.

Carefully read the labels:

For details on serving sizes, calories, and nutritional content, consult the nutrition labels.

Seek for items with low levels of artificial ingredients, harmful fats, and added sugars.

Browse the Periphery:

Try to stick to the perimeter of the grocery store when you shop, as here is where you'll usually find the dairy, whole grains, fresh produce, and lean proteins.

Purchases from the inner aisles should be avoided as they frequently include packaged and processed foods that are heavy in harmful fats and added sugars.

Purchase in Bulk (Non-Perishable Items):

To save costs and cut down on packaging waste, think about buying non-perishable goods like grains, beans, nuts, and seeds in large quantities.

To keep bulk goods fresh and stop them from spoiling, store them in airtight containers.

Think About Convenience Foods Carefully:

While convenience meals might save time, go for minimally processed foods that are low in sodium, bad fats, and added sugars.

Look for canned beans, frozen veggies without seasonings or sauces, and precut fruits and vegetables.

Respect Your Budget:

Establish a grocery budget and make an effort to keep to it by buying only necessities and avoiding impulsive buys.

To save money, think about using coupons, purchasing store-brand goods, or going shopping at discount retailers.

Be Adaptable and Flexible:

Be open to modifying your meal plan in response to shifting tastes, seasonal food, and product availability.

Make inventive use of leftovers to reduce food waste and expedite meal preparation.

You can choose better options, save time and money, and make sure your meals are filling and nutritious by using these helpful grocery shopping and meal planning ideas.

Frequently Held Myths Regarding Fad Diets and Superfoods

In the world of nutrition, fad diets and superfoods frequently create buzz and excitement, but they can also be accompanied by widespread misconceptions. The following are some myths about superfoods and fad diets:

Trendy Diets:

Rapid Weight Loss Fixes: A lot of fad diets promise quick weight loss by severely restricting or eliminating specific food groups. Although there is a chance of immediate weight loss, this type of diet is frequently not long-term sustainable and can result in vitamin deficiencies, muscle loss, and rebound weight gain if the diet is stopped.

One-Size-Fits-All Approach: Fad diets frequently advocate for a one-size-fits-all strategy that ignores the variations in each person's metabolism, way of life, and food preferences. What suits or is beneficial for one individual might not be for another.

Removal of Whole Food Groups: Some fad diets promote the removal of whole food groups, such as fats or carbs, which can result in nutritional imbalances and deficits in vital elements. Negative relationships with food and disordered eating behaviors can both be exacerbated by restrictive eating patterns.

Lack of Scientific Evidence: Many fad diets are based on anecdotal evidence, testimonials, or faulty research, but they rarely have scientific proof to back up their claims. Before adopting a diet, it is imperative to critically assess the veracity and trustworthiness of the claims made.

Focus on the Short Term: Fad diets frequently put the short term ahead of sustainability and long-term health. They might overlook crucial facets of general health, like exercise, stress reduction, and mental wellness.

Superfoods:

Superfoods are frequently touted as having extraordinary health advantages or as a panacea for a wide range of illnesses. Superfoods are not a replacement for a balanced diet and healthy lifestyle, even though some of them are high in nutrients and have health-promoting qualities.

Overemphasis on Individual Foods: The phrase "superfood" may give rise to the false impression that certain foods possess superpowers and can make up for unhealthy eating patterns or lifestyle choices. As part of a balanced diet, a range of nutrient-rich foods are actually what lead to optimal health.

Cost and Accessibility: People on a tight budget or residing in places where these foods are not easily accessible may find it difficult or costly to obtain certain superfoods. There is a vast array of reasonably priced and easily obtainable nutrient-rich dietary options.

Elimination of Other Nutrient-Rich meals: If one is just concerned with superfoods, they may neglect other nutrient-rich meals that have comparable health advantages. To guarantee a diet that is well-rounded and offers a wide range of nutrients, variety is essential.

False information and hype: The phrase "superfood" is frequently employed in marketing campaigns to generate buzz and increase sales. When evaluating the health benefits of superfoods, it's crucial to review claims made about them cautiously and take into account the whole context of a person's diet and lifestyle.

even if superfoods and fad diets could have certain advantages, it's crucial to approach them critically and with prudence. The greatest way to attain long-term health and well-being is to follow a balanced diet that prioritizes a range of nutrient-rich foods, frequent exercise, and smart lifestyle choices.

Consumption of Food and Mental Health

Nutrition affects mood control, brain function, and general well-being, all of which are important components of mental health. The following are some ways that diet may affect mental health:

Brain Function: For the brain to work at its best, it needs a constant flow of nutrients. The production of neurotransmitters, nerve signaling, and the development and repair of neurons are all aided by nutrients including omega-3 fatty acids, vitamins B6 and B12, folate, and antioxidants.

Mood Regulation: Studies have shown a correlation between enhanced mood regulation and a lower incidence of depression and certain nutrients, including omega-3 fatty acids, which are present in walnuts, flaxseeds, and fatty fish. The synthesis and metabolism of neurotransmitters like serotonin, which is involved in mood regulation, depend on other minerals like magnesium and zinc.

Chronic inflammation has been linked to the emergence of mood disorders, including anxiety and depression. Inflammation may be lessened and mental health may be supported by eating a diet high in anti-inflammatory foods, such as fruits, vegetables, whole grains, nuts, seeds, and fatty fish.

Gut-Brain Axis: New research indicates that mental health is significantly influenced by the billions of bacteria that live in the gastrointestinal system, or gut microbiota. A healthy gut microbiota is supported by a balanced diet high in fiber, probiotics, and prebiotics; this may have a good impact on mood and cognitive performance.

Blood Sugar Regulation: Mood and energy levels can be impacted by variations in blood sugar levels. Eating meals that are well-balanced in terms of proteins, carbs, and healthy fats helps control blood sugar levels and gives the brain a consistent supply of energy.

Micronutrient Deficiencies: An increased risk of depression and other mental health disorders has been associated with deficiencies in specific vitamins and minerals, including vitamin D, vitamin B12, iron, and folate. Maintaining mental health and preventing micronutrient deficiencies can be achieved by eating a diverse and nutrient-rich diet.

Hydration: Dehydration can affect one's emotions and cognitive abilities. Maintaining appropriate hydration and promoting general brain health require drinking enough water throughout the day.

Diet Quality: Studies indicate that following a healthy diet, like the DASH (Dietary Approaches to Stop Hypertension) diet or the Mediterranean diet, may reduce the risk of depression and improve mental health outcomes. These diets provide an emphasis on complete, minimally processed foods that are high in whole grains, fruits, vegetables, lean meats, healthy fats, and whole grains.

diet is very important for mental health and overall wellbeing. People can improve their mental health and lower their risk of mood disorders and cognitive decline by eating a balanced diet that is high in vital nutrients and supportive of gut health, controlling their blood sugar levels, and drinking plenty of water. Additionally, developing individualized nutrition plans to meet mental health goals can be facilitated by consulting with a registered dietitian or other healthcare provider.

Foods to Support Mental and Emotional Health

Because of their nutrient content and possible effects on brain health, a number of foods are recognized to promote mood and cognitive performance. Some meal examples that may improve mood and cognitive function are as follows:

Fatty Fish: Omega-3 fatty acids, especially EPA (eicosapentaenoic acid) and DHA (docosahexaenoic acid), are abundant in fatty fish, which include salmon, mackerel, trout, sardines, and herring. Omega-3 fatty acids have been connected to better mood, cognitive function, and a lower incidence of depression. They are crucial for the health of the brain.

Leafy Greens: Rich in folate, a B vitamin essential for neurotransmitter production, dark leafy greens such as spinach, kale, and Swiss chard are a great supply of this vitamin. A deficit in folate has been linked to a higher risk of depression and cognitive deterioration.

Berries: Antioxidants, such as flavonoids and anthocyanins, are abundant in berries, especially blueberries, strawberries, raspberries, and blackberries. These compounds have been related to enhanced cognitive performance and neuroprotective effects.

Nuts and Seeds: Packed with of antioxidants, omega-3 fatty acids, and other nutrients that promote brain health, nuts and seeds include walnuts, almonds, flaxseeds, chia seeds, and pumpkin seeds. Regular consumption of nuts and seeds has been linked to enhanced cognitive performance and a lower chance of age-related cognitive deterioration.

Whole Grains: Packed with fiber, vitamins, minerals, and antioxidants, whole grains such as oats, brown rice, quinoa, barley, and whole wheat promote cognitive function and brain health. It has been shown that eating whole grains as part of a balanced diet improves cognitive function and lowers the risk of cognitive impairment.

Legumes: Rich in fiber, protein, complex carbs, and vitamins that promote brain health are legumes, such as beans, lentils, chickpeas, and peas. They give the brain a consistent supply of energy and support stable blood sugar levels, both of which are critical for mood management and cognitive performance.

Avocados: High in monounsaturated fats that promote mental health and perhaps elevate mood, avocados are a great food choice. They also include vitamin E, an antioxidant associated with neuroprotection and improved cognitive function.

Dark Chocolate: Studies have indicated that the flavonoids and other antioxidants found in dark chocolate can elevate mood, lower stress levels, and improve cognitive performance. Eating dark chocolate in moderation that has a high cocoa content (at least 70%) may improve mood and cognitive function.

Curcumin, a substance with anti-inflammatory and antioxidant qualities found in turmeric, may enhance mental health and elevate mood. Supplementing with curcumin may help improve cognitive function and lessen the symptoms of depression, according to research.

Green Tea: Green tea has antioxidants called catechins that have been linked to better cognitive performance and a lower chance of age-related cognitive decline. Green tea's L-theanine and caffeine content may also improve mood, concentration, and focus.

CHAPTER FIVE

These nutrient-dense foods can improve mood and cognitive performance, boost brain health, and enhance general well-being when included in a balanced and varied eating pattern. To make sure you're getting a wide variety of nutrients that promote healthy brain function and mental health, it's critical to focus on a diversified selection of foods.

Recognizing Food Allergies and How They Affect Health

Food allergies arise from the immune system misinterpreting specific proteins in food as dangerous compounds and reacting inappropriately to them. Histamines and other substances are released as a result of this immunological reaction, causing symptoms that might be moderate or severe. A closer look of food allergies and their effects on health is provided below:

Frequent Food Allergens: Compared to other foods, some foods are more prone to trigger allergic reactions. The "Big 8," or the eight most prevalent food allergies, are as follows:

Milk

Eggs

Almonds

Tree nuts, including cashews, walnuts, and almonds

Soy

Wheat

Fish

Shellfish

Food allergies can cause a wide range of symptoms that can affect different sections of the body. Typical signs and symptoms include of:

Skin responses include edema, eczema, hives, and itching.

Symptoms of the digestive system: diarrhea, vomiting, nausea, or abdominal discomfort

Symptoms of the respiratory system include nasal congestion, wheezing, sneezing, and trouble breathing.

Heart palpitations, dizziness, or, in extreme situations, unconsciousness are signs of cardiovascular disease.

Anaphylaxis is a severe, perhaps fatal allergic reaction that can cause a variety of symptoms from several body systems and needs to be treated right away.

Diagnosis: A combination of the patient's medical history, physical examination, allergy testing (blood or skin prick tests), and oral food challenges carried out under a doctor's supervision are usually used to identify food allergies.

Effects on Health: The physical, mental, and overall quality of life of individuals with food allergies can all be significantly impacted. In order to prevent allergic responses, people with food allergies need to closely monitor their diet. This may entail reading food labels, inquiring about ingredients when dining out, and keeping emergency medication on hand in case of unintentional exposure (such as epinephrine auto-injectors).

Risk Factors: A family history of allergies, early exposure to allergenic foods, genetics, and other allergic disorders (such eczema or asthma) can all raise a person's chance of developing food allergies.

Management and Treatment: Strict avoidance of the allergenic food or foods that cause allergic responses is the main course of treatment for food allergies. Epipen users should promptly administer epinephrine (adrenaline) via an auto-injector (like an EpiPen) in the event of an accidental exposure or severe allergic reaction. Food allergy sufferers should collaborate closely with medical professionals to create a personalized management plan that comprises emergency procedures, dietary recommendations, and continuous observation.

Potential for Allergy Prevention: There are a few ways to prevent food allergies in infants and early children, such as avoiding needless dietary restrictions during pregnancy and infancy, introducing allergenic foods early and frequently (in consultation with a healthcare provider), and exclusively breastfeeding for the first six months of life.

All things considered, food allergies are a severe health issue that need to be carefully managed, supported, and educated about. Food allergies do not yet have a cure, but improvements in medical care and research give those who suffer from them hope for better results and a higher quality of life.

The Advantages of Batch Cooking and Meal Planning

For people and families, meal planning and bulk cooking have several advantages, such as:

Time savings: By arranging your meals for the week ahead of time, meal planning helps you to expedite the cooking process. Cooking in bulk, or producing a large amount of food at once, can cut down on the amount of time spent in the kitchen during hectic workdays. You may spend more time on other activities and less time cooking during the week if your meals are planned and prepared in advance.

Cost Savings: By minimizing food waste, avoiding impulsive purchases, and taking advantage of promotions and discounts, meal planning and bulk cooking can help you save money. Eating out or buying pre-packaged convenience foods can be more expensive than cooking at home or buying supplies in bulk.

Better Eating Practices: Arranging your meals ahead of time enables you to choose foods with greater consideration and purpose. A well-balanced diet that satisfies your nutritional demands can be achieved by include a range of nutrient-dense foods in your meal plan. In addition, batch cooking gives you the freedom to choose healthier cooking techniques like baking, steaming, or grilling and to regulate portion proportions.

Decreased Stress: By removing the last-minute rush to decide what to have for supper, meal planning helps to cut down on stress and decision fatigue. Having a meal plan in place will help you feel more structured and organized, which will make it simpler to adhere to your nutritional priorities and goals.

Enhanced Variety: When you plan your meals ahead of time, you can include a wider range of items in your diet, such as new recipes, seasonal vegetables, and cuisines from different cultures. You can make more distinct recipes in larger quantities with batch cooking, which increases your weekly menu options.

Portion Control: By dividing meals into individual servings through batch cooking, you may more easily regulate portion sizes and prevent overindulging. Meals that have been preportioned can also be easily packed for lunches or taken on the go.

Convenience: It's simple to get a healthy meal when you're pressed for time or energy when you have pre-prepared meals on hand. Preparing meals ahead of time can be quite helpful, especially if you're returning home from work late or simply need to grab a quick bite before leaving.

Family bonding: Organizing meals and preparing in bulk can be cooperative family activities. Planning meals, grocery shopping, and cooking together as a family can promote shared responsibility for one another's health and wellbeing as well as communication and teamwork.

All things considered, meal planning and batch cooking are useful strategies for encouraging better eating habits and family unity while also saving time, money, and stress. You can reap the benefits of increased peace of mind when it comes to food choices and more effective meal preparation by implementing these tactics into your daily routine.

Time-Saving Recipes and Ideas for Meal Prep

You may simplify your cooking routine and make it easier to consume wholesome meals throughout the week by using time-saving meal prep ideas and recipes. To get you started, consider these suggestions and recipes:

Ready-to-eat ingredients:

Clean and cut up veggies: Ready-to-eat veggies, such as bell peppers, carrots, broccoli, and cauliflower, can be kept in resealable bags or containers for quick use in omelets, stir-fries, and salads.

Cooking grains and legumes: Make large quantities of rice, quinoa, lentils, or beans ahead of time and keep them chilled or frozen. Soups, casseroles, grain bowls, and salads can all be made with cooked grains and legumes as the foundation.

Vegetables: Roasting veggies can improve their flavor and make them easier to include in meals all week long. Examples of these vegetables are sweet potatoes, Brussels sprouts, and squash.

Prepared Morning Meals:

Overnight oats: In a jar or container, combine rolled oats, milk or yogurt, chia seeds, and your preferred toppings (fruit, nuts, and spices). Place it in the fridge for the entire night to make a simple and quick breakfast.

Egg muffins: In a muffin tin, whisk together eggs, cheese, cooked protein (such sausage or ham), and vegetables. Once baked, place the egg muffins in the freezer or refrigerator for a portable, high-protein breakfast.

Cooking Proteins in Bulk:

Baked chicken breasts: After seasoning with your preferred herbs and spices, bake the chicken breasts in the oven until they are cooked through. Throughout the week, you may use shredded chicken in salads, wraps, sandwiches, and soups.

Pull pork prepared in a slow cooker: Prepare a big quantity of pulled pork in a slow cooker using your preferred spice or barbecue sauce. For quick and tasty meals, try the pulled pork in tacos, salads, and grain bowls.

Prepare lunches in advance:

Mason jar salads: Arrange items in layers within the jars, including lush greens, veggies, grilled chicken or chickpeas for protein, almonds, seeds, and vinaigrette. Just shake the container to combine everything just before eating.

Burrito bowls: Fill separate containers with cooked grains, beans, roasted vegetables, cheese, salsa, and guacamole. Serve cold or reheat in the microwave for an easy and filling lunch alternative.

Fridge-friendly Recipes:

Soups and chilis: Make big pots of these and divide them into individual freezer-safe containers. For a hearty and filling dinner, reheat in the microwave or on the stove.

Pasta bakes, lasagnas, and casseroles can be prepared in advance and frozen for later use. For a quick dinner option, thaw in the fridge overnight and bake until heated through.

Snack Bundles:

For easy-to-graze snacks throughout the week, divide up foods such as nuts, seeds, dried fruit, cheese cubes, and sliced veggies into separate containers or resealable bags.

In a big bowl, combine nuts, seeds, dried fruit, and dark chocolate chips to make your own trail mix. Trail mix can be portioned out into tiny bags or containers for a quick and filling snack.

You can streamline mealtime, save time and money, and enjoy tasty and nourishing meals all week long by implementing these time-saving meal prep ideas and recipes into your daily routine. Don't be afraid to experiment with different flavors and combinations, and feel free to modify the recipes and ingredients to fit your dietary requirements and preferences!

Overcoming Typical Obstacles to Eating Healthfully

Making nutritious food choices a regular part of your lifestyle might be difficult at times, but with the appropriate approaches, you can get beyond typical roadblocks and enjoy a healthier diet. The following are some typical obstacles to eating healthily, along with solutions:

Time Restrictions:

Challenge: Finding time to plan and cook healthy meals can be challenging for people with busy schedules.

Solution: To save time during the week, give meal preparation and bulk cooking top priority. Make time every week to organize your meals, make a shopping list, and prepare ingredients ahead of time. On weekends or days off, prepare a big batch of food and portion it into individual containers for convenient warming during the week.

Quick-to-cook foods:

Problem: When you're pressed for time or energy, convenience foods like frozen dinners, packaged snacks, and fast food are frequently available and tempting to grab for.

Solution: Keep a supply of simple yet wholesome foods in your home, like canned beans, whole grain bread, pre-cut veggies, and low-sodium canned soups. When you're in a hurry, go for healthier convenience foods like microwaveable whole grain rice, single-serve Greek yogurt, and prepackaged salads.

Social Coercion:

Problem: Maintaining a healthy diet can be difficult when attending social events, parties, and eating out with friends and family.

Solution: To avoid overindulging in unhealthy foods, have a healthy lunch or snack before heading out to social gatherings. Look for healthier options on restaurant menus, and don't be hesitant to request dietary-specific adjustments or substitutes. Give more thought to the company you keep than just the food.

Emotional Consumption:

Challenge: Cravings for comfort foods heavy in sugar, fat, and calories can be brought on by stress, boredom, melancholy, and other emotions.

Solution: Rather than eating in response to feelings, adopt mindful eating by observing signs of hunger and fullness. Look for other strategies to manage your stress and emotions, such taking a walk, deep breathing exercises, or doing something you love. Stock up on nutritious snacks so you can satiate your cravings without going off your plan.

Food Spending Cap:

Budget-friendly healthy eating can be difficult, particularly when lean meats and fresh produce can be more expensive than packaged and processed foods.

One possible solution is to organize your meals around less expensive foods such as whole grains, beans, lentils, eggs, and frozen fruits and vegetables. When feasible, purchase in bulk and take advantage of special offers and discounts. For reasonably priced, locally grown produce, think about purchasing at farmers' markets or enrolling in a community-supported agriculture (CSA) program.

Absence of Cooking Ability:

Challenge: It can be difficult to produce wholesome meals at home if you don't have a lot of cooking experience or culinary skills.

Solution: Begin with basic recipes and work your way up to more complex ones over time. To broaden your horizons, try different flavors, ingredients, and cooking methods. Attend cooking classes, study online guides, or get help from friends and relatives. Keep in mind that cooking is a skill that gets better with experience.

Impractical Expectations:

Challenge: Feelings of frustration and disappointment might result from setting extremely stringent or unreasonable objectives for healthy eating.

The answer is to make attainable goals that fit your priorities, tastes, and way of life. Rather than trying to completely alter your diet all at once, concentrate on making tiny, long-lasting improvements to your eating habits. Honor your accomplishments and treat yourself with kindness when you encounter obstacles or disappointments.

You can establish a balanced and long-lasting approach to nutrition that promotes your general health and well-being by identifying and resolving typical barriers to eating healthfully. Never forget that altering your eating habits for the long term requires consistency, tolerance, and determination.

Handling Food Cravings and Emotional Eating

Creating healthier coping mechanisms for emotions and cravings is a necessary step in overcoming emotional eating and food cravings. The following advice can assist you in controlling your food cravings and overcoming emotional eating:

Determine Triggers:

Keep an eye out for the feelings, circumstances, and ideas that set off your cravings or cause you to overeat emotionally. Stress, boredom, melancholy, loneliness, and social circumstances are common triggers.

Engage in Mindful Eating:

Pay attention to your body's signals of hunger and fullness, and eat in a focused, distraction-free manner. Take your time, enjoy every bite, and pay attention to the food's flavor, texture, and sensory aspects.

Consider if you're eating for emotional reasons or because you're actually hungry before you eat. Look into alternate non-food ways to deal with your emotions if you're not physically hungry.

Look for Other Coping Strategies:

Create a toolkit of substitute coping strategies to handle stress and emotions without turning to food. This may be journaling, taking a stroll, doing deep breathing exercises, listening to music, or partaking in a favorite pastime or activity.

Try out many methods to determine which ones are most effective for you, then make them a part of your regular routine as constructive coping mechanisms.

CHAPTER SIX

Respond to Emotional Needs:

Take the time to determine and attend to the underlying emotional needs rather than utilizing food as a narcotic or diversion from difficult emotions. If you're having trouble coping with challenging feelings or situations, ask friends, family, or a therapist for assistance.

Make self-care a priority and give attention to things that feed your mind, body, and soul, such getting adequate sleep, working out frequently, and spending time with close friends and family.

Maintain a Food Journal:

Maintain a food diary or notebook to record your cravings, feelings, and eating patterns. This might assist you in tracking your development over time and in identifying emotional eating behaviors and triggers.

Make use of your food journal to evaluate your eating patterns and pinpoint areas that require work. Honor your accomplishments and draw lessons from whatever obstacles or failures you face.

Keep a stock of healthier alternatives:

Stock your house with nutritious snacks and substitutes for the foods that set you off. To satiate cravings without throwing off your diet, go for nutrient-dense foods like fruits, vegetables, nuts, seeds, yogurt, and whole grains.

When enjoying snacks, remember to eat mindfully and in moderation. To avoid overindulging, don't eat straight from the packet.

Seek Assistance:

Seek out understanding, accountability, and support from friends, family, or a support group. It can make you feel less alone and more supported on your path if you talk to others about your issues with emotional eating and food cravings.

Think about seeking the specialized advice and assistance of a licensed dietitian, therapist, or counselor who specializes in emotional eating.

Treat Yourself with Kindness:

When you give in to cravings or moments of emotional eating, treat yourself with kindness and gentleness. Acknowledge that every day presents a fresh chance to make healthy decisions and that it's natural to experience periodic setbacks.

As you work toward kicking emotional eating and forming healthy habits, remember to be kind to yourself, forgive yourself, and concentrate on making progress rather than perfection.

You may learn to deal with emotional eating and control your cravings for food in better ways by putting these tips and tactics into practice. Remind yourself that overcoming emotional eating requires time, patience, and practice. However, with perseverance and support, you can enhance your general wellbeing and cultivate a better connection with food.

Encouragement and Assistance for Readers to Keep Eating Healthfully

It's crucial to keep in mind that every step toward healthier eating, no matter how tiny, is a win to be celebrated for people who are starting down this path. Here are some words of wisdom and inspiration to keep you inspired to follow a healthy diet:

Celebrate Your Progress: Give yourself a time to reflect on and be grateful for the progress you have already achieved. Any positive adjustment you make is a step in the right direction, whether it's cooking more regularly at home, adding more fruits and vegetables to your meals, or finding healthier substitutes for your favorite snacks.

Concentrate on the Positive: Rather of focusing on mistakes or setbacks, pay attention to the constructive adjustments you've made and the healthy routines you've established. Accept that obstacles will inevitably arise along the way, and seize the chance to grow stronger and learn from your experiences.

Be Kind to Yourself: As you negotiate the ups and downs of eating a healthy diet, remember to treat yourself with love and self-compassion. Show yourself the same compassion, tolerance, and understanding that you would show a friend going through a similar ordeal.

Establish Achievable and Realistic Goals for Yourself: Considering your own tastes, way of life, and situation, establish attainable goals for yourself. Divide more ambitious objectives into more doable, smaller steps, and acknowledge each accomplishment as it occurs.

Discover What Works for You: Try out various strategies for eating healthily to see which ones work best for you. Find the techniques that work for you and your lifestyle, whether it's meal planning, bulk cooking, mindful eating, or discovering healthier alternatives for your favorite foods.

Remain Consistent: Maintaining a healthy diet over time requires consistency. Even on the days when you're not as motivated or life gets hectic, stick to your priorities and goals. Recall that over time, modest, persistent efforts can result in substantial advancement and long-lasting transformation.

Seek Support: Encircle yourself with like-minded others who share your dedication to eating healthily, whether they are friends, family, or online communities. In trying times, rely on them for support, accountability, and inspiration.

Practice Gratitude: Develop an attitude of thankfulness for the healthful foods you can eat and the chance to make decisions that will improve your health. Every day, take a time to acknowledge how many nutrient-dense foods you have access to and the advantages they have for your body and mind.

Remain Inspired: Continue to be inspired and driven by exploring new culinary methods, recipes, and advice on maintaining a balanced diet. Keep your meals interesting and fun by following cookbooks, social media accounts, and blogs about healthy eating.

Remember Your Why: Whether it's to feel more invigorated, elevate your mood, maintain your long-term health, or just to savor tasty and healthy foods, go back to the reasons you decided to make eating healthily a priority. As a source of inspiration and drive for your quest, never lose sight of your why.

Above all, keep in mind that progress, not perfection, is what healthy eating is all about. Accept the adventure with open arms and a readiness to change, grow, and learn as you go. You have the ability to reach your health objectives, and every decision you make for your wellbeing is a significant step in the direction of a better, healthier life.

Summary

In summary, adopting a healthier diet is a personal, continuous effort that calls for commitment, tolerance, and self-compassion. You may improve your physical and mental health as well as your general quality of life by making wholesome foods a priority, engaging in mindful eating, and maintaining balance in your diet and lifestyle.

It's critical to keep in mind that progress, not perfection, is what healthy eating is all about. Establish attainable objectives, acknowledge your accomplishments, and take lessons from any obstacles or failures you face. No matter how tiny, every wise decision you make improves your general health and wellbeing.

When assistance is needed, ask friends, family, and medical experts for it. You should also surround yourself with a community of people who share your dedication to leading a healthy lifestyle. Always remember to treat yourself with kindness, cultivate thankfulness for the nourishing foods in your life, and stay motivated by trying out new recipes, cooking methods, and nutritious eating advice.

In the end, adopting a healthy diet is a worthwhile adventure that can change your life from the inside out. You can achieve your health objectives and lead the greatest possible life if you approach the road with an open mind and a desire to learn and grow. Cheers to your ongoing good health, joy, and overall wellbeing.

THE END